Get Rid Of Warts

The Ultimate Guide To Getting Rid Of Warts

By: Heather Rose

TABLE OF CONTENTS

PUBLISHERS NOTES

DEDICATION

This book is dedicated to those having low self-esteem because of warts.

INTRODUCTION

Warts are seen on children as well as on adults. They can be on very visible areas, like the face and hands. They are quite embarrassing to have and sometimes impossible to cover with a bandage. They can grow on complicated places like on finger joints or in between the legs.

When playing a sport or at work it is easy to hurt and bleed them, being quite painful at times. Even though they are not considered dangerous they are quite bothersome and embarrassing to have.

Many have tried the different treatments we will describe below. Some have been successful but most have had a recurrence of the warts and even more. For many it has been very costly, very painful and frustrating, therefore, we want to share with you a powerful and effective natural remedy that has removed my warts forever.

As a child, I suffered first hand with this terrible condition. I had warts on my knuckles, hands and between my legs. My mother would try everything there was possible, first she tried over the counter products with no success. The warts continued to multiply and grow. Then the dermatologist suggested the liquid nitrogen which actually froze each wart. It was so painful but I was able to support the pain, I guess the humiliation of having warts was even harder to take. The warts fell off, but they came back in a short time. My mother did not know what else to do, because she felt that it was not worth putting me through the pain again, especially with a method that proved not to be permanent.

Then one day a family doctor noticed my hands and how big my warts were. The doctor told my mother he knew about a very old remedy they use in Spain. He told her: "Just Believe Me! It will work!" And it did... after three applications the warts where totally gone.

Keep reading and you will find out exactly how we did it and why this healing substance is so powerful.

CHAPTER 1- TALKING ABOUT WARTS

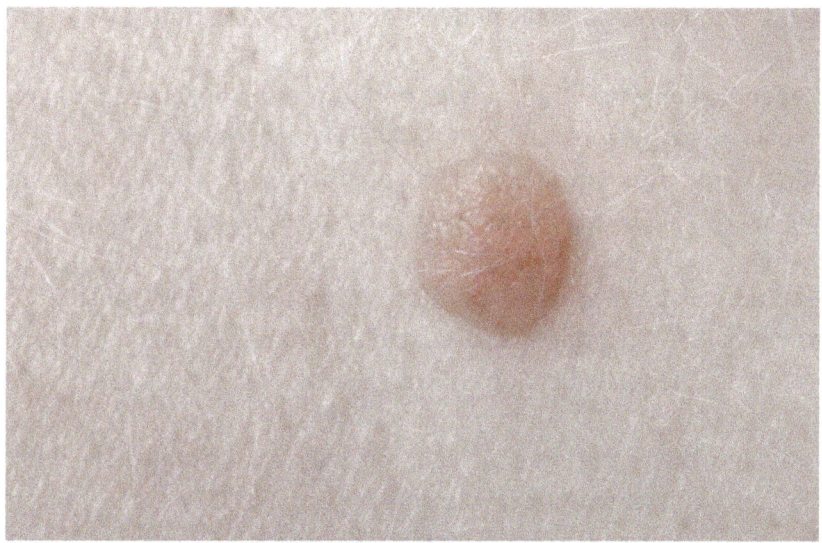

A wart is generally a small, rough growth, typically on hands and feet but often on other locations, that can resemble a cauliflower or a solid blister. They are caused by a viral infection, specifically by human papillomavirus 2 and 7. Any skin surface of the body is susceptible to forming the cauliflower-like appearance which are essentially benign tumors on the skin.

Warts are most often transmitted from person-to-person contact. If you touch a wart on someone else it is possible that you can grow a wart as well. It is possible to get warts from others; they are contagious. If contact is made with broken skin, it increases the likelihood substantially. They are also passable via inanimate objects such as bath towels and other objects that might have come in contact with the wart and allow for it to be passed.

There are many varieties of warts with the most common being considered largely harmless. Some of them may typically disappear after a few months but others can last for years and can recur.

Types of Warts

There are several different types of warts. The common wart is the one you would most often find on your hands and fingers. There are also plantar warts or foot warts which can be found on the soles of the feet, normally under the surface of the skin.

Depending on where they are located, these can have a debilitating impact on a person's ability to walk. Flat warts are flat on their surface and often grouped in large numbers. They can be found on the legs, of adult females mostly, or the faces of small children.

Genital warts are one of the most common sexually-transmitted diseases (STD) out there, and treated differently, for the most part, than the other classifications of warts.

Although there are several common ways warts are dealt with, Genital warts should not be treated with any of these methods. They could cause you serious harm and damage.

Please reserve these common remedies only to warts on your feet, hands, legs and other non-genital regions. If you want to treat genital warts, your best bet is to consult with your doctor.

Some warts will eventually go away on their own, although doctors do not seem to know why this happens. It may take months or years, but some warts simply disappear one day never to be seen again. Others require treatment to deal with them and make them go away. Even if a wart is not causing you physical pain or discomfort, it is a good idea to look at treating them. Just having the warts can allow them to spread and infect other parts of your body as well as infect other people

CHAPTER 2- MEDICAL TREATMENTS

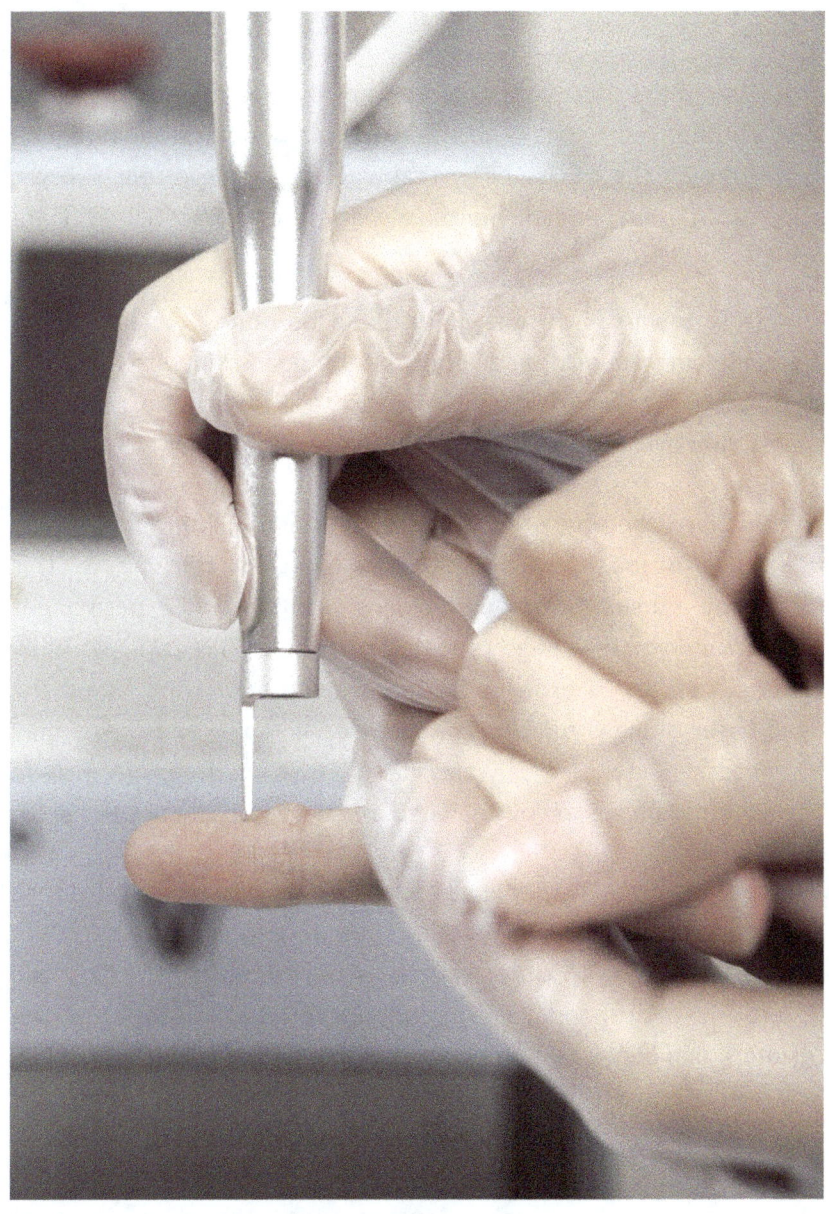

If you have stubborn warts and home treatment isn't helping, your doctor may suggest one of the following approaches, based on the location of your wart, the degree of your symptoms and your preferences. Doctors generally start with the least painful, least destructive methods, especially in young children.

Medical Procedures

Acid: One of the most common methods is to burn warts off with a mild acid applied topically to the wart. Many applications may be required over the course of several weeks to achieve this. Salicylic acid, cantharidin, and dichloroacetic (or trichloroacetic) acid are useful.

Removing a wart with salicylic acid can be done by cleaning the area, applying the acid, and removing the dead skin with a pumice stone or emery board. It may take up to 50 weeks to remove a wart. Other acid methods may be used.

Freezing (cryotherapy, or liquid nitrogen therapy). Your doctor may use liquid nitrogen to destroy your wart by freezing it. This treatment is usually very painful and is often not a permanent solution and you may need repeated treatments. Freezing works by causing a blister to form under and around your wart. Then, the dead tissue sloughs off within a week or so. Local anesthesia may be necessary for large warts, and risks of freezing include permanent damage to your nail bed and nerves in the treated area.

Cantharidin. Your doctor may use cantharidin — a substance extracted from the blister beetle — on your warts. Typically, the extract is mixed with other chemicals, painted onto the skin and covered with a bandage. The application is painless, but the resulting skin blister can be uncomfortable and may cause swelling. However, the blister has an important purpose. It lifts the wart off your skin, so your doctor can remove the dead part of the wart.

Minor surgery. This involves cutting away the wart tissue or destroying it by using an electric needle in a process called electrodessication and curettage. However, the injection of anesthetic given before this surgery can be painful, and the surgery may leave a scar. For these reasons, surgery is usually reserved for warts that haven't responded to other therapies. Note: The excision of warts is not recommended since the surgery may leave a painful scar and it is common for warts to return in the scar tissue.

Laser surgery. Laser surgery can be expensive, and it may leave a scar. It's usually reserved for tough-to-treat warts. New technology has enabled doctors to use lasers to destroy the wart. The procedure, performed in the physician's office, is expensive and is likely to result in some scarring. Its efficacy in comparison to other destructive approaches in unproven.

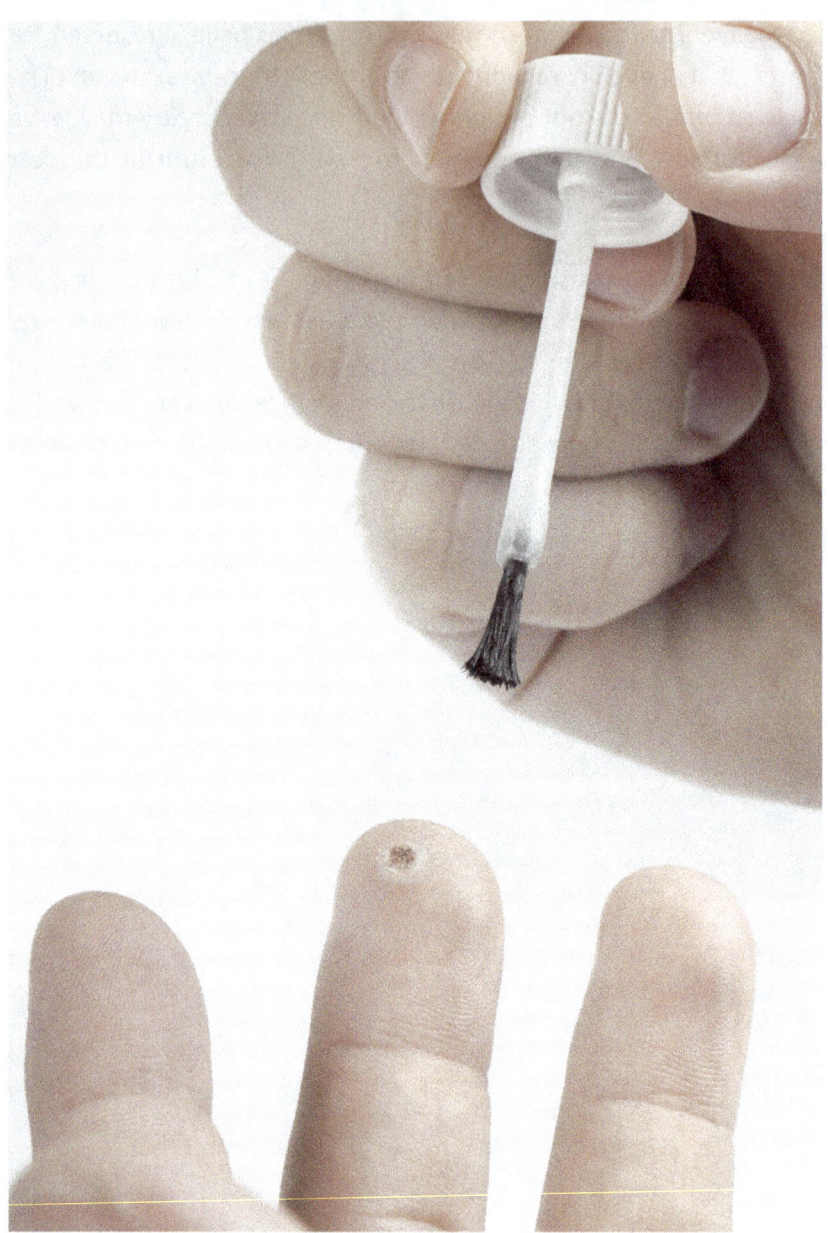

Prescription Medications

If you have a bad case of warts that hasn't responded to standard treatments, your doctor may refer you to a dermatologist for further treatment, including:

Immunotherapy. This type of treatment attempts to harness your body's natural rejection system to fight off warts. Topical immunotherapy medications that may be prescribed for stubborn warts include squaric acid dibutylester and a gel called imiquimod (Aldara). Imiquimod is marketed for the treatment of genital warts but has also proved effective for treating common warts. However, warts may return when these therapies are stopped.

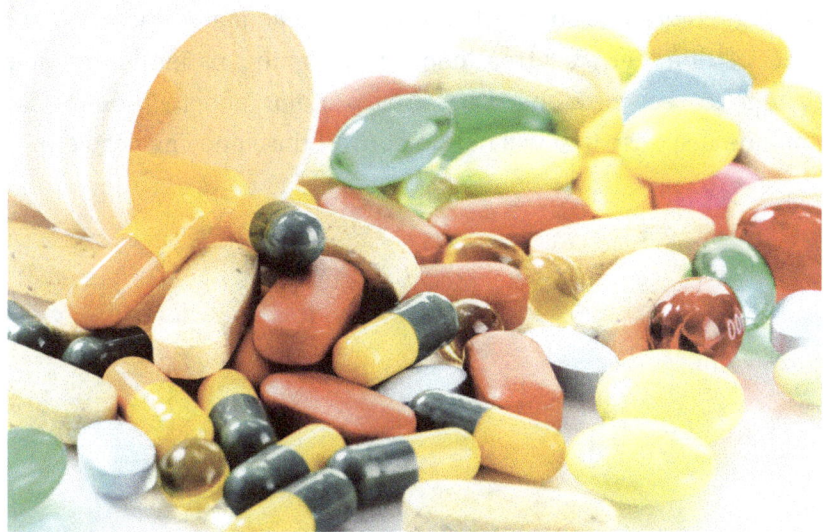

Bleomycin (Blenoxane). Your doctor may inject a wart with a medication called bleomycin, which kills the virus. Bleomycin is used with caution for warts, but in higher doses, is used to treat some kinds of cancer. Risks of this therapy include nail loss and damage to the skin and nerves.

Retinoids. Derived from vitamin A, these medications disrupt your wart's skin cell growth. Your doctor may prescribe a retinoid cream or an oral medication. These medications make your skin extra sensitive to the sun, so be sure to protect your skin from the sun while taking them.

Common warts can be tough to get rid of completely or permanently, especially when they appear around and under your nails. And, if you're susceptible to the wart virus, you probably always will be. New warts may crop up even after a successful treatment. More than one treatment may be necessary to manage the problem. Warts are viral, and antibiotics are not effective for viral illnesses.

There are many other treatments available for the treatment of warts.

No single therapy is so effective that it has eliminated the use of all others. Ultimately, all treatments rely on the patient's immune system to recognize the wart virus proteins and to produce an immune response that will rid the body of this annoying problem.

CHAPTER 3- COMMON NATURAL REMEDIES

When you begin treating a wart be aware that depending on the size and type it is, it can take weeks to get rid of – sometimes months. If you experience progress with a treatment, keep at it and be patient. Plenty of times a wart will just disappear on its own (as your body builds up immunity against the virus). You can read the most common natural remedies below or you can go straight to discover the most powerful and simple way to get rid of warts within days, further down this book.

Before applying a remedy, wash wart area clean with soap and water then pat dry with a clean towel. Also wash hands with soap and water before handling remedy and touching the wart. Wash hands again after applying treatment to prevent further infection.

General Natural Treatments

1. Apple Cider Vinegar: Saturate a cotton ball with apple cider vinegar (ACV) and apply to wart, secure in place with a Band-Aid or tape. Do this every night before bed, remove in the morning. Good for all warts, recommended especially for Plantar and flat warts.

2. White Household Vinegar & Baking Soda: Sprinkle a heavy coat of baking soda on the wart then drizzle vinegar over it. Do this once in the morning and once at night until wart is gone.

3. Band-Aids Or Tape: Known as the duct tape treatment, keep the wart wrapped tight in tape (without cutting off circulation) 24/7 until it disappears. Band-Aids, duct tape, packing tape and scotch tape will all work with the same results. Change the tape daily.

4. Baking Soda: Make a thick paste of baking soda and water, apply to wart and cover with tape or a Band-Aid.

5. Clear Nail Polish: Paint the wart with a coat of clear nail polish, reapply as needed until wart is gone.

6. Hydrogen Peroxide: Apply to wart each day using a cotton swab.

7. Toothpaste: Dab regular toothpaste generously on top of the wart then cover with a Band-Aid. Do this daily until wart is gone.

8. Aspirin: Rub wart with olive oil then place an aspirin tablet on top and secure with a piece of tape or Band-Aid. Change daily. Or crush an aspirin tablet fine then add a few drops of water to make a paste. Apply to wart and cover with a Band-Aid. Watch on sensitive skin.

9. Vitamin C Tablet: Crush the Vitamin C tablet fine then make a paste with water. Apply to wart and wrap it with tape or a Band-Aid to secure. Change daily.

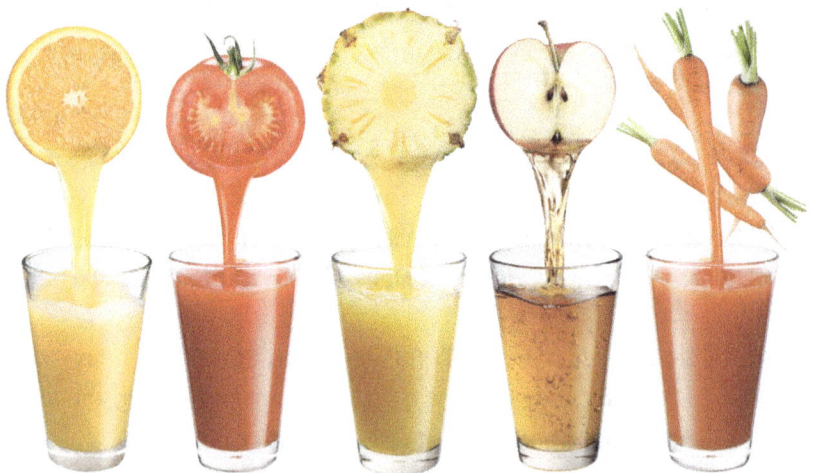

Fruits and Vegetable Treatments

1. Potatoes: Cut a potato in half and rub the potato juice over the wart.

2. Lemons: Rub a slice of lemon over the wart for 5 minutes twice a day. You can also dab lemon juice directly on the wart.

3. Limes: Rub a slice of freshly cut lime over the wart for 5 minutes twice a day. You can also dab lime juice directly on the wart.

4. Bananas: Cut a piece of banana skin just bigger than the size of the wart. Place the peel white side down on top of the wart then cover with tape or a Band-Aid to hold in place. Replace daily until wart is gone. You can also rub the wart with a fresh slice of banana.

5. Eggplant: Cut a thin slice of eggplant just a bit larger than the wart and hold in place with a piece of tape or Band-Aid. Change daily until wart has disappeared. Good remedy for children or those with sensitive skin.

6. Onion: Rub a slice of freshly cut onion over the wart twice a day.

You can also sprinkle onion slice with salt first then apply to wart

Another suggested treatment is to drizzle lemon juice on the wart then cover with a freshly cut piece of onion (wrap a piece of tape or Band-Aid around to hold in place).

7. Carrots: Grate a fresh carrot then mix with olive oil until you have a thick paste. Apply to wart and cover with a Band-Aid. Do this twice a day until wart disappears.

8. Apples: Apply a freshly cut slice of apple to the wart and secure in place with tape or a Band-Aid. Change twice a day until wart is gone.

9. Garlic: A few variations of this treatment: Crush garlic then cover the wart completely with the garlic, wrap tape or a Band-Aid to secure in place. Do this every night before bed. Apply the juice of garlic to the wart twice a day. Each night at bedtime apply a slice of garlic to the wart, wrap with a bandage.

10. Figs: Mix mashed fig with a bit of olive oil and apply to wart, cover with a Band-Aid. Do this daily until wart is gone.

11. Radishes: Cut a slice of radish just the size of the wart, cover the wart and secure in place with a Band-Aid. Change daily.

12. Pineapple: Apply a freshly cut piece of pineapple to the wart morning, noon and night until wart is gone.

Oil and Extract Remedies

1. Witch Hazel: Rub Witch Hazel into the wart a couple times a day.

2. Clove Oil: Mix a few drops of clove oil with olive oil then apply to wart, change daily.

3. Vitamin E Oil: Rub into wart then cover with a Band-Aid, do this three times a day.

4. Vitamin A Oil: Rub into wart then cover with a Band-Aid, do this three times a day.

5. Garlic Capsule Oil: Rub into wart then cover with a Band-Aid, do this once in the morning and cover with a Band-Aid.

6. Castor Oil: Rub Castor Oil into the wart a couple times each day until wart is gone, cover with a Band-Aid. You can also mix baking powder or baking soda and castor oil into a paste and apply to wart, cover with a bandage. Change daily.

7. Grapefruit Seed Extract: Apply a few drops to the pad of a

Band-Aid then cover wart, change daily.

8. Oil of Oregano: Mix a few drops with olive oil then apply to the pad of a Band-Aid–cover wart and change daily.

9. Lavender Essential Oil: Carefully dab the wart with a drop of Lavender EO, cover with a Band-Aid. Do this once a day.

10. Geranium Essential Oil: Mix a few drops with olive oil then apply to the pad of a Band-Aid–cover wart and change daily.

11. Lemon Essential Oil: Mix a few drops with olive oil then apply to the pad of a Band-Aid–cover wart and change daily.

12. Tea Tree Oil: (also known as Melaleuca Oil) Dab the wart two times a day with tea tree oil until wart disappears. Cover with a Band-Aid during the day, remove Band-Aid at bedtime.

13. Frankincense: Apply a drop directly to the wart and cover with tape or a Band-Aid. Change Band-Aid daily. Reapply drop of Frankincense twice a week.

14. Vegetable Oil: Smother the wart with a thick coat of vegetable oil then apply tape or a bandage. Do this each night before bed and first thing in the morning.

Herbs and Plant Treatments

1. Dandelions: Apply dandelion milk from the stem of a dandelion to the wart. Cover with tape or a Band-Aid. Apply two times a day until wart is removed.

2. Aloe Vera: Apply the gel from an aloe vera plant to the wart then top with a cotton ball and Band-Aid. Change twice a day until wart is gone.

3. Basil Leaves: Crush fresh basil leaves and cover the wart, then secure in place with a Band-Aid.

4. Marigolds: Break open marigold leaves and apply the plant juice directly to wart. Do this daily until wart is gone.

5. Milkweed: A Native American wart remedy is to rub the milk from a milkweed plant into the wart several times a day until wart has been removed.

Wart Soaks

Soaking the warts daily in treated baths will help soften them and help the warts respond to treatment. Can also help fight the virus and prevent infection.

Soaking treatments are also worthwhile doing before sloughing the skin with an emery board or pumice stone. Soak wart daily in a warm bath of baking soda and water.

1. Soak wart daily in a hot bath of Epsom salt and water.

2. Soak wart in very hot water until it becomes lukewarm (do this daily, don't have the water so hot it burns you though). Plain hot water is fine but you can also add some vinegar.

Wart Immunity Boosters

Beef up your immunity system so your body can fight the wart virus internally. Here are a few suggested immunity boosters I have on hand that are recommended for fighting warts.

1. Cabbage: Eat a lot of fresh, raw cabbage each day.

2. Garlic: Add fresh, chopped garlic to your food whenever possible.

You can also take garlic pills or capsules daily.

3. Limes: Squeeze fresh lime juice over food or add fresh lime juice to a glass of water and drink this twice a day.

4. Broccoli: Eat fresh, raw broccoli daily.

5. Oranges: Eat an orange once a day.

6. Bananas: Good for potassium, eat one a day to fight warts.

7. Onions: Top everything suitable with chopped fresh onion, preferably raw but cooked is fine too.

This information is simply a collection of home remedies for getting rid of warts – not professional medical advice. Please seek a doctor's opinion when unsure or to confirm appropriate treatment for your wart.

CHAPTER 4- AN ODD REMEDY

If you thought you had heard it all, think again. Let me now urge you not to get disgusted and take this information with utmost seriousness because you will be amazed with the healing properties that this viscous substance holds.

But before we go any further, let me ask you the following: Have you ever heard about the controversy regarding stem cell research?

Advocates like Christopher Reeve, Michael Fox and even Nancy

Reagan shouted its cause. And no, it is not stem cells that we will use to cure warts, please keep reading.

The controversy comes from the use of aborted fetuses for the purposes of research. While I highly doubt that many women would ever undergo an abortion in order to produce stem cells for research, the religious right argued that their use in stem cell research was immoral and that federal funding for such research should be disallowed. In fact, they believe that such stem cell research shouldn't be performed.

My feelings are that the procedure should be safe, legal, and extremely, extremely rare. That being said, I couldn't see why a naturally aborted embryo should be relegated to mere biohazard status when it could possibly be used for research to save or improve the human life of someone who has already been born.

It turns out that there are other alternative methods of procuring stem cells for research. One of those alternative methods is through the use of human placenta and also through the use of menstrual blood.

Yes you heard it right, women's menstrual blood; or as I like to call it 'healing menstrual blood'. This exact healing substance is our powerful natural remedy to get rid of warts forever.

Here's how researchers are harvesting this fluid, (you are NOT going to have to do this for your use of it in the removal of warts, I just want you to understand the great significance that menstrual blood has for medical research). To store menstrual blood for future research a woman inserts a cup shaped like a tampon into her vagina on her heaviest flow day for approximately 3 hours in order to preserve a specimen of 10 to 20 milliliters of blood. That is then poured into a container and shipped back to a lab to be used or stored for future use.

As I understand it some women are paying a fee of $499 and then an additional $99 per year to store their own menstrual blood for future use. The stored cells can be thawed and used to help in the treatment of breast cancer, stroke, Alzheimer's disease, Parkinson's or any one of a number of possible future health problems for the patient or for a beloved family member.

That's the selling point, anyway. I wonder if anyone will ever think to so conveniently package a storage method for women who just wish to donate menstrual blood in order to help others. A woman has an average of 500 periods in her lifetime. That's a lot of stem cells from just one woman.

Imagine if you convinced as many women to harvest menstrual blood as the women who donate blood to the Red Cross annually. How many people could benefit from stem cell's curative properties? How much progress could be made towards research to find a cure for life threatening diseases? And the best part is that I can't think of a single moral or ethical issue that anyone could come up with for not using the stem cells gathered from menstrual blood or umbilical cords from full term pregnancies.

I doubt this will ever catch on like wildfire because of people's initial gross out factor. However, it's not as though anyone is asking for someone to ingest actual menstrual blood in order to facilitate healing. The stem cells are extracted from "processed" menstrual blood. It's kind of cool to know that it's an option, storing menstrual blood to harvest stem cells, that is. Instead of women throwing their period out with the trash, they could use it to preserve or improve someone's life.

That someone might even, someday being themselves.

If it indeed, women's menstrual blood can be helpful in the treatment of cancer and other serious illnesses, wouldn't it just make sense to believe that this same substance can have the powerful healing properties to eliminate warts as well? I certainly know this is absolutely true, because it worked for me.

I hope you have gotten an idea of the rich healing properties contained on this powerful women's menstrual blood substance. And though the idea may be unpleasant for some, it may not be as unpleasant as having a body covered with repulsive warts.

Method of Application

The method of application is very simple indeed. You are going to put a rich drop of menstrual blood on a Band-Aid or bandage and wrap each wart with it. Yes! You read it correctly! That is all it takes. A drop of menstrual blood on a bandage the size of the wart, if multiple warts are to be targeted, then use several Band-Aids; if a large wart is targeted then use a larger bandage. Apply it before bed and leave it on throughout the night. The next morning, remove the Band-Aid and rinse or shower the treated area. Repeat this for several nights.

Results may start to show within three applications.

Although this healing substance may be very accessible for some people (especially for women between the ages of 13 and 53) It may not be so for others, especially for men; In which case it is recommended to seek the collaboration of a very close female family member or friend. In most of the cases the blood can be harvested from a mother (as it was in my case when I was only nine years old), a sister, or a wife.

NOTE: Always verify first that the donor has tested negative for any viral diseases before applying menstrual blood from another person onto your own warts.

Conclusion

I know that for some of you, the thought of this remedy may cause you to be grossed out, but let me tell you that the procedure to do it is so simple and straight forward, and the results so incredibly accurate that you will not regret it a bit.

I was only a child when I got treated with this remedy and had no idea of what the blood was. I would only say "the magical Band-Aids DID IT!" I never knew what they contained until I was older. All I knew was that the warts were totally gone FOREVER! It did not hurt and they left no scars either. And it was totally FREE!

For years I have passed this remedy on to others that have the same problem and I have heard many success stories where their warts were gone forever as well in a matter of only days.

If you are currently suffering from warts on your body, I really hope that you can believe the powerful healing properties contained on menstrual blood. I truly hope that you take this amazing step and experience this remarkable remedy to really get rid of your warts once and for all. And I absolutely wish you many blessings in your years to come free of warts forever.

ABOUT THE AUTHOR

Heather Rose is an expert for both physical and mental health with years of practice to back it up. From her own experience of working with those who are experiencing the parenting problems of various degrees, she now shares her knowledge of dealing to a large audience.

She writes on various strategies on managing individuals with such problems and how to help their lives more enjoyable and much less stressful and frustrating. It also makes life easier for the family and the people around them cope with their symptoms.